CHAPTER LEADER'S GUIDE TO

Patient Rights

Practical Insight on Joint Commission Standards

Jean S. Clark, RHIA, CSHA

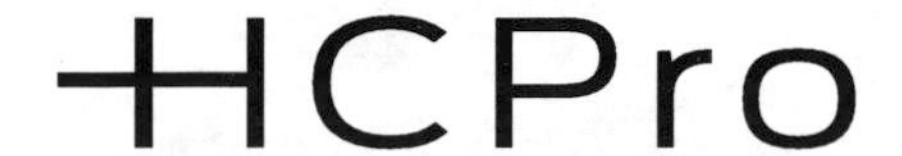

Chapter Leader's Guide to Patient Rights: Practical Insight on Joint Commission Standards is published by HCPro, Inc.

 5 4 3 2 1

Download the additional materials of this book at *www.hcpro.com/downloads/9141.*

ISBN: 978-1-60146-811-6

Jean S. Clark, RHIA, CSHA, Author
Jaclyn Beck, Editor
Mike Briddon, Executive Editor
Emily Sheahan, Group Publisher
Mike Mirabello, Senior Graphic Artist
Matt Sharpe, Production Supervisor
Shane Katz, Art Director
Jean St. Pierre, Senior Director of Operations

HCPro, Inc.
75 Sylvan Street, Suite A-101
Danvers, MA 01923
Telephone: 800/650-6787 or 781/639-1872
Fax: 800/639-8511
E-mail: *customerservice@hcpro.com*

Visit HCPro online at: *www.hcpro.com* and *www.hcmarketplace.com*

03/2011
21867

Contents

About the Author

Jean S. Clark, RHIA, CSHA

Jean S. Clark, RHIA, CSHA, is the director of accreditation at Roper Saint Francis Healthcare in Charleston, SC, and is currently a member of the Joint Commission Hospital Advisory Council. Clark has served on The Joint Commission (JCAHO) Standards Review Task Force and the expert panel for the Information Management chapter, which resulted in sweeping changes for the accreditation process beginning in January 2004. A past president of the American Health Information Management Association (AHIMA), she received AHIMA's Distinguished Member Award and the Volunteer Award. She is the past president of the International Federation of Health Records Organizations (IFHRO). She is the contributing editor to *Medical Records Briefing,* and author of seven editions of *Information Management,* five editions of *Ongoing Records Review,* the *HIM Director's Guide to Recovery Audit Contractors,* and the first edition of *The HIM Directors' Handbook,* all from HCPro, Inc.

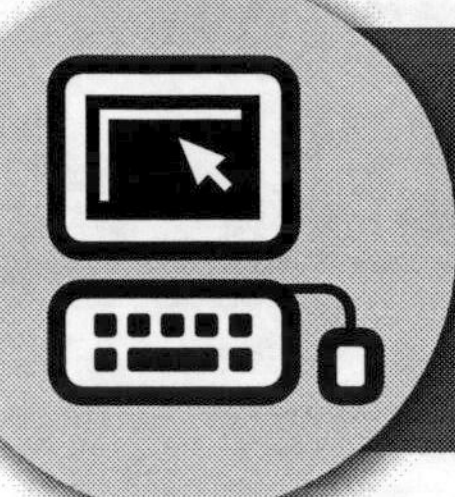

DOWNLOAD YOUR MATERIALS NOW

Sample tools and documents from this book, including a special PowerPoint® presentation to help readers communicate these materials with their staff, are available online at the website listed below. This is an additional service provided by HCPro, Inc., and the authors of our *Chapter Leader's Guide* series.

www.hcpro.com/downloads/9141

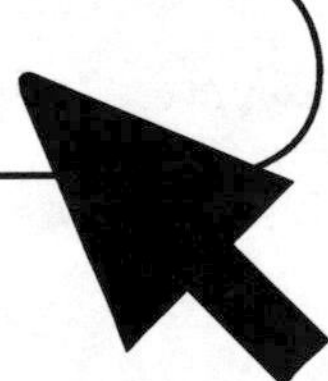

Thank you for purchasing this product!

HCPro

PART 1

Patient Rights in the Organization

The standards contained in the Rights and Responsibilities of the Individual chapter (sometimes informally called the patient rights chapter) focus on developing and communicating patient rights, participation in care decisions, informed consent, right-to-know care providers, end-of-life issues, and personal rights and services provided by the organization to respect patient rights. The patient rights chapter also outlines the responsibilities patients have with regard to care and treatment.

Today, patients are much better informed with regard to their health and welfare. Resources about disease processes and treatment care choices are abundant on the Internet. Gone are the days when the patient feels reluctant to question or discuss his or her care with doctors or other caregivers.

Only when patients understand their illness and what types of care, treatments, and services can be provided will they be able to make good decisions about care. For example, a brief discussion of a surgical procedure will not provide the patient with the necessary information for him or her to make good decisions about whether to have a procedure. It is important to obtain an informed consent that outlines the risks, benefits, and alternatives that enable the patient to make sound decisions affecting his or her unique situation. End-of-life decisions can also be difficult for families if there is no advance directive to express the patient's wishes if recovery is not an option, and the individual absolutely has the right to make his or her own decisions about healthcare and to clearly understand the available options. The only way to do this is to adhere to the tenets of the patient rights chapter!

Figure 1.1 lists the direct impact of these standards.

How Does This Chapter Affect the Organization as a Whole?

Communication is the key! It becomes the hospital's duty to provide an atmosphere of respect and open communication with patients from the minute they are present for care and treatment. It is everyone's job to encourage patient participation by informing patients of their rights, providing avenues for participation in their care, and establishing a partnership between the patient and the caregivers. For example, during daily rounds, the physician or nurse can ask patients if they have questions about their care, or to clarify things that they do not understand. A bulletin board should be posted in the patient's room that identifies the caregiver on duty that day to promote open communication. It is also important to continually ask patients if they have any questions every time new information is given to them.

1.1 Rights and Responsibilities of the Individual (RI) Direct Impact Standards List

RI.01.01.03–The right to be informed

EP1 – Information is provided in a manner tailored to the patient's age, language, and ability to understand

EP2 – Language interpreting and translation services are provided

EP3 – Information is provided to patients who have vision, speech, hearing, or cognitive impairments

RI.01.02.01–The right to participate in decision-making

EP1 – The patient is involved in making decisions about his or her care and the right to have his or her own physician promptly notified

EP3 – The right to refuse care is respected

EP6 – Surrogate decision-makers can be involved in decisions when the patient is unable to make decisions

EP7 – Surrogate decision-makers have the right to refuse care on the behalf of the patient

RI.01.03.01–The right to give or withhold informed consent

EP7 – Informed consent includes a discussion about the patient's proposed care

EP9 – Informed consent discussion includes potential benefits, risks, and side effects; the likelihood of achieving goals; and any potential problems

EP11 – Informed consent discussion includes reasonable alternatives and any risks, benefits, and side effects of alternatives

RI.01.05.01–The right to make end-of-life care decisions

EP3 – Advance directive policies are implemented

EP13 – Advance directives are honored

RI.01.06.03–The right to be free of neglect, exploitation, or abuse

EP2 – All allegations, observations, and suspected cases of neglect, exploitation, and abuse that occur in the hospital are evaluated

EP3 – Allegations, observations, and suspected neglect, exploitation, and abuse are reported to the appropriate authorities

Some patients may feel reluctant to ask questions of their caregivers, so it is up to the hospital to provide an atmosphere that encourages transparency and open communication. Other patients may be more comfortable communicating, and this openness should never be discouraged. The more caregivers know about the patient, the better the care decisions will be. And in many cases, the patient will recover faster and follow instructions once he or she is at home. It just makes sense: The more you know, the better the care, resulting in a more compliant patient who follows instructions to full recovery.

Patients also have responsibilities, and it is the hospital's job to fully explain what these are and in such a way that the patient can understand. Understanding rights and accepting responsibilities makes for an empowered patient. Empowered patients feel in control of their destiny, so to speak. They will open up more about how they are feeling. They will feel respected and begin to feel as part of the team, not just a body in the bed to be poked at and prodded. Empowered patients become informed patients, and a sense of trust builds between the patient and caregivers, which promotes quality care and safety for the patient.

Needless to say, this chapter affects every aspect of care, from the admitting office to the discharge nurse and physician. Not only will the patient need to be informed of his or her rights and responsibilities, but so will every member of the patient care team.

What Is the Impact on Leadership and Administration?

Leadership and administration set the tone for the patient rights chapter and must "walk the talk." If patient rights are not clearly understood from the top down then no training, brochures, or education will ever create a true sense of patients as partners in their care, treatment, and services. Employees must hear it from senior leadership (and this includes medical staff leadership) that providing patient care, treatment, and services in a transparent and collaborative way **IS** the culture of the organization in partnership with the individual patient.

Creating a culture that is transparent and collaborative with patients may take some work on the part of leadership. Here are a few suggestions that senior leadership can use to establish, support, and foster a culture of transparency and collaboration:

- Incorporate this philosophy into the hospital's mission statement
- Clearly state the philosophy in the patient handbook (usually provided on admission or at the time of outpatient services)
- Understand the patient's rights and responsibilities
- Enable senior leadership to be easily accessible to patients, staff, and management
- Establish a process to write thank-you notes to patients
- Use multidisciplinary rounding (including physicians) in the patient room
- Keep the family involved
- Conduct open forums with patients
- Conduct regular patient satisfaction surveys and ask questions related to this type of culture (See Figure 1.2 for a sample patient satisfaction survey.)

1.2 Patient Satisfaction Survey

Question	Yes	No
1. Were you provided with a copy of the hospital's patient rights and responsibilities?		
2. Were they explained to you in a way you could understand?		
3. Were your caregivers, including physicians, introduced to you by name and job responsibility?		
4. Were you asked if you had an advance directive, such as a living will or healthcare power of attorney?		
5. Were you treated with respect and dignity?		
6. Were you informed of the process to voice a complaint?		
7. Were you informed of how to contact The Joint Commission?		
8. If you had surgery or a procedure, were the risks, benefits, and alternatives explained to you?		
9. Overall, do you feel you were encouraged to participate in decisions regarding your care, treatment, and services?		

Additional comments:

____

____

____

Who Owns the Requirements of the Patient Rights Chapter?

Shared ownership between all members of the healthcare team is essential for compliance with the requirements of this chapter. Because healthcare is so complex and its details are so interrelated, ownership must be shared. For example, if the registration department does not see advance directives as part of their job to inquire at the time of registration, it may never be known that the patient has a document that expresses his or her end-of-life wishes. Nurses need to share this responsibility by validating the existence of an advance directive during the initial nursing assessment. The health information management department needs to make sure the document is part of the medical record. This same scenario can be carried out in the operative area with regard to informed consent.

It is important to understand that the patient has ownership when it comes to healthcare as well, and is often not even aware that a better informed healthcare team can provide better care and treatment. The previous section outlined some ways to get the patient involved in a team approach to care and treatment.

Remember, when it comes to the rights of the individual as outlined in the patient rights chapter, you cannot assume someone else is going to get the job done. The patient rights chapter could be considered more cross-functional as far as ownership is concerned than the other chapters because the processes required for compliance cover more than one department. Identifying key roles within the organization is helpful for understanding this chapter.

The Role of the Board

The board must understand the importance of respecting patients' rights with involvement in their care and treatment. The board should make it clear that each patient, regardless of his or her personal values, beliefs, and preferences will be treated with dignity, respect, and as an individual. If this can be built into the board's mission and vision, then it sets the tone for the rest of the organization to follow.

The Role of the Senior Leaders

It is the responsibility of the senior leaders to educate the board and others with regard to the requirements of this chapter and to ensure through policy and practice that patients' rights are carried out throughout the organization. Senior leaders will also have to be prepared to deal with breaches in patients' rights and be willing to take responsibility when processes fail to meet the standards set for the organization. This could also involve the legal department of the organization, an ethics committee, human resources, and other departments dealing directly with patient care. It is also the responsibility of leadership to ensure that patients and their families understand their responsibilities with regard to "ownership" of their care and treatment, and provide mechanisms for informing the patient in a way the patient can understand. This will include budgeting dollars for supporting the right people and the right tools to keep patients informed.

The Role of the Medical Staff

Because medical staff are always on the frontline of patient care, they also must be well-educated with regard to patient rights. Make patients' rights and the medical staff's responsibilities part of orientation and continuing education for the medical staff. Some organizations have medical staff applicants sign a "creed" or "standards of behavior" as part of the application process. Medical staff leaders will have to be willing to deal with physicians who do not respect patients' rights. The Bylaws of the Medical Staff should not only outline what is expected of physicians, but also what happens when a breach occurs.

An example of a creed might read something like this:

- *I promise to inform my patients and their families about their illness, the treatment options, and any risk and benefits in a manner they can understand.*

- *I promise to be open to my patients concerns and deal with them in a proper manner.*

- *I promise to inform my patients when incidents occur.*

- *I promise to respect the wishes of my patients with regard to their care and treatment.*

The Role of the Clinical Staff and Others

In their various roles, nurses, physical therapists, housekeepers, and billing staff, just to name a few, serve patients on a daily basis. The hospital may have patient representatives whose specific focus is patients' concerns with regard to care, treatment, and rights. But, it is important to remember that such concerns are everyone's job, and the better educated each member of the healthcare team is with regard to patients' rights and responsibilities, the better patients' experiences will be.

The Role of the Patient

As previously stated, patients need to be informed that they have the right to the following:

- Effective communication

- Participation in their care

- Informed consent (See Appendix C for a sample informed consent form)

- Knowing their caregivers

- Participation in end-of-life decisions

- Personal rights
- Services provided by the organization to respect their rights

It is just as important for the patient to know their responsibilities as well. These responsibilities include the following:

- **Providing information about their health conditions**
  - The patient can be prompted during the physician history and physical and during nursing assessments and reassessments
  - Consultants and other caregivers such as dieticians, physician therapists, and/or the chaplain can also encourage the patient to provide information
- **Asking questions**
  - Caregivers should take every opportunity to encourage questions from patients and family. Daily rounding is a good way to do this. Routine visits from patient representatives and even administration can provide an atmosphere conducive to encouraging patients to ask questions about their care.
- **Following instructions**
  - Each caregiver should stress the need to follow instructions. Using a teach-back method to determine patient understanding is a good way to ensure instructions are understood. Easy to read pamphlets and follow-up instruction sheets are another way to communicate discharge instructions and follow-up care.

- **Being respectful of staff**
  - A respectful staff is the example that must be set by the caregivers; however, it should be made clear (if the occasion arises) that patients should also show respect to their caregivers. A process should be in place to deal with unruly patients and families.
- **Meeting financial responsibilities**
  - Generally, registration staff are involved in explaining the patient's financial responsibility. The patient handbook is also a good place to provide this information and who to contact with any questions they may have.

How to meet and maintain the rights of the patient, as well as the patient's responsibilities, will be discussed later in this book. However, Figure 1.3 provides a grid that outlines the key players' responsibilities by standard and element of performance. It should be noted that hospitals may differ in who is responsible for different aspects of the elements of performance and the grid should be used as a guide. The "M" under "Other" refers to the required measure of success if an element of performance receives a requirement for improvement at the time of a survey.

Figure 1.4 defines a communication plan for specific patient rights and duties that are traditionally assigned to certain departments and individuals. It gives a suggested outline of when and how chapter leaders should communicate patient rights and responsibilities to each department or individual.

1.3 Rights and Responsibilities of the Individual and Key Players Outline

Standard and Element of Performance	The Governing Board	Senior Leaders	Medical Staff	Clinical Staff	Other Hospital Staff	The Patient	Other	Documentation Required
RI.01.01.01 Respects, protects, and promotes patient right								
EP 1 Written policies	X	X	X	X	X			Policy
EP 2 Informing the patient of rights and responsibilities			X	X	X			
EP 4 Treating the patient with dignity and respect	X	X	X	X	X		M	
EP 5 Effective communication			X	X	X	X	M	
EP 6 Respecting cultural and personal values, beliefs, preferences	X	X	X	X	X	X	M	
EP7 Rights to privacy			X	X	X		M	
EP8 Pain management			X	X	X	X		
EP9 Religious and other spiritual services			X	X	X	X	M	
RI.01.01.03 Receiving information in a way the patient understands								
EP1 Tailored to age, language, and ability to understand			X	X	X	X	M	
EP2 Providing interpreting and translation services		X	X	X	X		M	
EP3 Communicating effectively with regards to vision, speech, hearing or cognitive impairments		X	X	X	X		M	
RI.01.02.01 Rights to participate in decisions regarding care, treatment, and services								
EP1 Notifying physician immediately								

1.3 Rights and Responsibilities of the Individual and Key Players Outline *(cont.)*

EP2 Written information about the right to refuse care				X	X			Written information re: right to refuse care, treatment, services
EP3 Right to refuse care in writing to the patient			X	X	X			
EP6 Rights for a surrogate decision-maker when patient is unable to make decisions	X	X	X	X	X	X		
EP7 Rights of the surrogate decision-maker is respected	X	X	X	X	X			
EP8 Involvement of the family in care decisions to the extent permitted by patient or surrogate decision maker			X	X	X	X	X (e.g., Family	
EP20 Patient and surrogate decision-maker provided with information about the outcomes of care								
EP21 Patient and surrogate decision-maker provided information about unanticipated outcomes of care that relate to TJC identified sentinel events			X	X	X			
EP22 Licensed, independent practitioner responsible for the care informs the patient of unanticipated outcomes of care	X	X	X					
RI.01.03.01 Right to give or withhold informed consent								
EP1 Required policy outlines	X	X	X	X	X			Policy
EP2 Care, treatment, and services that require informed consent			X	X				
EP3 Exceptions to informed consent			X	X				
EP4 Process to obtain informed consent			X	X				

1.3 Rights and Responsibilities of the Individual and Key Players Outline *(cont.)*

Standard and Element of Performance	The Governing Board	Senior Leaders	Medical Staff	Clinical Staff	Other Hospital Staff	The Patient	Other	Documentation Required
EP5 Documentation in the medical record			X	X	X (e.g., HIM Director			
EP6 When a surrogate decision maker may give consent			X	X				
EP7 Content related to proposed care, treatment, and services			X					
EP9 Benefits, risks, side effects, achieving goals, problems with recuperation			X					
EP11 Alternatives			X					
EP12 When information must be discussed or disclosed			X	X				
EP13 Emergency situations			X	X			M	
RI.01.03.03 Give or withhold informed consent to produce or use recordings, films, other images for purposes other than care								
EP1 Obtains informed consent from patient for use other than care	X	X	X	X		X		Policy
EP2 Documentation of informed consent and recordings, etc., are to be used			X	X	X			Documentation of use
EP3 Inability to obtain consent, production may occur if according to policy established through ethical mechanism	X	X	X	X	X		Ethics Com-mittee	

1.3 Rights and Responsibilities of the Individual and Key Players Outline *(cont.)*

EP4 Product remains in hospital's possession until patient's permission is obtained		X	X	X	X	X		
EP5 If consent not obtained, production is destroyed, or nonconsenting patient is removed from production			X	X	X			
EP6 Patient is informed of right to request cessation of production			X	X	X			
EP7 Confidential statement signed by any not bound by hospital policy							X (e.g., Film crew)	Signed confidentiality policy
EP8 Patient can rescind consent			X	X	X	X	M	
RI.01.03.05 Research, investigation, and clinical trials								
EP1 Hospital reviews all research protocols and weighs risks and benefits			X	X	X			
EP2 Information provided to patient (e.g., purpose, duration, description, benefits, risks, discomforts and side effects, advantageous alternative care)			X	X	X			
EP3 Refusal will not jeopardize care			X	X	X			
EP4 Research consent form documents information to make decision to participate			X	X	X	X	M	Informed consent
EP5 Patient informed that refusal has no bearing on care			X	X	X	X		Informed consent
EP6 Name of person providing information and date form is signed			X	X	X	X		Informed consent

1.3 Rights and Responsibilities of the Individual and Key Players Outline *(cont.)*

Standard and Element of Performance	The Governing Board	Senior Leaders	Medical Staff	Clinical Staff	Other Hospital Staff	The Patient	Other	Documentation required
EP7 Consent describes patient's rights to privacy, confidentiality, and safety			X	X	X	X		Informed consent
EP9 All information given to patient is kept in medical record			X	X	X	X	M	Medical record
RI.01.04.01 Patient's right to receive information about the person responsible for care and those providing care								
EP1 Patient is informed of the name of the physician, clinical psychologist, or other practitioner primarily responsible for care			X	X	X		M	
EP2 Patient is informed of the name of the physician, clinical psychologist, or other practitioner providing care			X	X	X		M	
RI.01.05.01 End-of-life decisions								
EP1 Written policies related to advance directives, forgoing or withdrawing life-sustaining treatment, and withholding resuscitative services	X	X	X	X	X			Policy
EP4 Define if advance directive will be honored for outpatient services	X	X	X	X	X			
EP5 Advance directives are implemented			X	X	X		M	

1.3 Rights and Responsibilities of the Individual and Key Players Outline *(cont.)*

EP6 Patient provided with written information about advance directives, withdrawing life-sustaining treatment, and withholding resuscitative services			X	X	X		M	Written information for example patient handbook, admitting information, brochures
EP8 On admission, patient provided with information on extent hospital is able, unable, or unwilling to honor and advance directive				X	X		M	
EP9 Documents whether patient does or does not have advance directives			X	X	X		M	Documents in medical records
EP10 Provides assistance if patient wishes to formulate an advance directive				X	X		M	
EP11 Those involved in care are aware of whether patient has an advance directive			X	X	X		M	
EP12 Patient's right to formulate, review, or revise advance directive is honored			X	X	X			
EP13 Hospital honors advance directives according to law, regulations, and hospital capabilities	X	X	X	X	X			
EP15 Documentation regarding patient's wishes concerning organ donation			X	X	X		M	Documents in medical record
EP16 Hospital honors patient's wishes concerning organ donation			X	X			M	
EP17 Existence or lack of advance directive does not determine patient's right to access care			X	X				

1.3 Rights and Responsibilities of the Individual and Key Players Outline *(cont.)*

Standard and Element of Performance	The Governing Board	Senior Leaders	Medical Staff	Clinical Staff	Other Hospital Staff	The Patient	Other	Documentation required
EP19 In outpatient settings, policy on advance directives is communicated to patients			X	X	X		M	
EP20 In outpatient settings, patients are referred to resources for assistance with formulating advance directive				X	X		M	
EP21 Deemed status only: How permission to obtained and documented is defined			X		X			
RI.01.06.03 Patient is free from neglect; exploitation; and verbal, mental physical, and sexual abuse								
EP1 Hospital determines how patients will be protected from neglect, exploitation, and abuse during care	X	X	X	X	X			
EP2 All allegations, observations, and suspected cases of neglect, exploitation, and abuse are investigated			X	X	X			
EP3 All of the above are reported to authorities based on evaluations			X	X	X			

1.3 Rights and Responsibilities of the Individual and Key Players Outline *(cont.)*

RI.01.06.05 Environment preserves dignity and contributes to a positive self-image								
EP2 Hospital settings providing longer term care (> 30 days) consider the number of patients assigned to a room (e.g., age, developmental levels, clinical conditions, diagnosis needs, hospital goals)				X	X		M	
EP4 Use of personal possessions and clothing				X	X		M	
EP15 Offers telephone and mail service				X	X		M	
EP16 Offers access to private telephones if patient requests				X	X		M	
EP17 Restricting visitors, mail, telephone calls, or other forms of communication must be made with the participation and family, if appropriate				X	X	X		
EP18 Any restrictions as noted in EP17 must be documented in the medical record			X	X	X		M	
EP19 Any restrictions as noted in EPs 17 and 18 must be evaluated for therapeutic effectiveness			X	X	X		M	
RI.01.07.01 Patient and family complaints must be reviewed								
EP1 Complaint resolution process is established	X	X	X	X	X			
EP2 Patient and family are informed about the process				X	X	X	M	

1.3 Rights and Responsibilities of the Individual and Key Players Outline *(cont.)*

Standard and Element of Performance	The Governing Board	Senior Leaders	Medical Staff	Clinical Staff	Other Hospital Staff	The Patient	Other	Documentation Required
EP4 Hospital resolves complaints if possible			X	X	X	X	M	
EP6 Patient is notified when complaint cannot be resolved immediately and follows up					X	X	M	
EP7 Phone number and address needed to file a complaint with state authority are provided to the patient					X	X	M	
EP10 Patient has right to voice complaints and recommend changes freely			X	X	X	X		
EP18 Deemed status – Patient is provided a written notice of decisions related to complaints to include name of hospital contact person, steps taken in investigation, results, date completed process			X	X	X		M	
EP19 Deemed status – Time frames are established for review and response		X			X			Written notice of decisions
EP20 Deemed status – Process for resolving complaints includes a timely referral of patient concerns about quality of care and premature discharges to the quality improvement organization (QIO)		X			X			
RI.01.07.03 – Rights to protective and advocacy services								
EP1 Patients needing protective services are provided resources to family and the courts				X	X			

1.3 Rights and Responsibilities of the Individual and Key Players Outline *(cont.)*

EP2 List of names, addresses, and telephone numbers of advocacy groups is maintained				X	X			Up-to-date lists maintained and available
EP3 Advocacy list given to patient when requested				X	X			
RI.01.07.07 – <u>For psychiatric hospital settings with stays over 30 days</u>, patients rights are protected if they work for or on behalf of the hospital								
EP1 Written policy		X						Policy
EP2 Policy is implemented				X	X		M	
EP3 Wages paid to patients are in accordance with law and regulations		X			X			
EP4 Work preformed by the patient is incorporated into the plan of care			X	X			M	
EP5 Patients have the right to refuse work		X			X			
RI.02.01.01 Patient responsibilities								
EP1 Written policy		X	X	X	X			Policy
EP2 Hospital informs patient about his or her responsibilities		X			X			

1.4 Patient Rights Communication Plan

To:	By:	What:	When:	How:
Board	Chapter Captain	Overview and Board's Role	First Board meeting of each year during triennial cycle	PowerPoint® presentation
	Chapter Captain	Board's Role	During quarter when survey is expected	PowerPoint presentation and handout
Medical Staff	Chapter Captain	Overview and doctor's role	First MEC/year	PowerPoint presentation
	Chapter Captain	Standards and EPs	Monthly MEC meetings	PowerPoint presentation
	Chapter Captain	Pertinent topics, for example informed consents; new information	As needed	Doctor newsletter, intranet site
Nurses	Chapter Captain or RN member of team	Standards, results of mock surveys, results of periodic performance review (PPR), nursing's role in compliance	Monthly or quarterly nursing leadership meetings, unit meetings	PowerPoint presentations, seminars, intranet site for The Joint Commission, newsletter
Staff	Chapter Captain or other member of team	Standards, results of mock surveys, results of PPR, staff roles	Monthly or quarterly department meetings, managers' meeting	PowerPoint presentations, seminars, intranet site for The Joint Commission, newsletter
Leadership	Chapter Captain	Overview, leaders' roles, PPR and mock findings	Quarterly	PowerPoint presentation

PART 2

Communication and Impact of Patient Rights

Part 1 provided a high level overview of the patient rights chapter, the impact on leadership and administration, and outlined who owns the patient rights chapter. This section of the book will focus on those individuals who need to carry out the requirements of the chapter, suggestions for who should be the chapter leader and their role, examples of how the chapter leader designates responsibilities, and how communication should be provided to hospital caregivers, other staff, and the patient and family.

Getting Organized

To be successful at the time of survey, you must be well-organized in a way that enables continuous survey readiness at all times. This means establishing a Joint Commission team whose responsibilities will be to:

- Conduct the annual periodic performance reviews for each chapter
- Conduct mock surveys

- Perform record reviews (or delegate this duty to the HIM [health information management] department)
- Ensure that policies are up-to-date and in compliance with standards
- Provide education and training
- Compile required documents for the time of the survey
- Identify and track deficiencies to resolution

It is usually the responsibility of the accreditation director or coordinator to establish and lead the team by assigning chapters and responsibilities, facilitating meetings of the team, and reporting deficiencies to senior leadership. Although everyone in the organization must take ownership in the success of a survey, it is unrealistic to think The Joint Commission will be on the top of everyone's mind. That is why a Joint Commission team has to be established: to keep Joint Commission compliance in the forefront of others' minds.

So who might the accreditation director consider as good candidates to lead the patient rights chapter? Consider the following individuals:

- **Patient representatives:** These individuals already work closely with patients and families, and may already have responsibilities to ensure information is provided in a way the patient or family understands. Patient representatives usually facilitate resolution of complaints and serve as the patient advocate. They may also assist in formulating advance directives.

- **Risk managers:** These individuals may also assist in resolving complaints and may understand the importance of informed consent and advance directives. They usually facilitate resolution of sentinel events.

- **RNs responsible for education to patient and family:** These individuals may develop patient educational tools and facility health literacy programs that would be beneficial to them in a chapter leader role.

- **HIM directors:** These individuals understand confidentiality and privacy for the patient. They are experts in documentation in the medical record as well as legal aspects of the record, and are well-informed with regard to advance directives, informed consent, and other aspects of patient rights.

- **Registration directors:** These individuals are first-line contacts with patients. They may be responsible for developing the patient handbook and often have the big picture in mind with regard to this chapter.

Duties of the Chapter Captain

The chapter captain should be responsible for the following:

- Scoring the chapter and providing input to the accreditation director to complete the periodic performance review (PPR). (See Figure 2.1 for an example of a completed annual PPR, with suggested action plans to improve compliance.)

- Developing education and/or educational tools and/or providing input to those responsible for education

2.1 Sample Annual Periodic Performance Review (PPR) Results

All standards and elements of performance are in compliance for the year except for the following with action plans:

Standard/EP	What?	Who?	Completion Date	Comments
RI.01.01.01, EP 7 – Privacy A category	Observed during mock tracer that patients were left in public hallways waiting for outpatient procedures.	Chapter team member to work with department managers to locate patients in private areas.	Within one week of notification (include specific date)	
RI.01.01.01, EP 9 – Religious and other spiritual services C category with measure of success	Not all requests by patients were being honored.	Chapter captain to work with pastoral care and nursing leadership to ensure documentation in medical record indicates patient wishes and that these are carried out. Audit medical records to ensure compliance.	30 days	
RI.01.02.01, EP 13 – Informed consent C category with measure of success	Informed consent was not being obtained in the endoscopy unit.	Endoscopy unit manager to put process in place to obtain informed consent prior to any procedure. Audit medical records to ensure compliance.	Within one week	

- Developing policies/procedures and/or providing input to ensure compliance with elements of performance requiring policies
- Developing tracer tools
- Conducting tracers, identifying and reporting noncompliance, resolving issues identified during tracers

Figure 2.2 provides a checklist of responsibilities for the chapter captain to complete.

Communicating With Physicians and Staff

You can have the best policies and procedures in the world, but if communication and understanding by those who need to know is not available, the intent of the patient rights chapter will never come to fruition. The chapter captain assigned to patients' rights, with guidance from the accreditation director, should develop a communication plan to ensure that everyone in the organization understands his or her roles and the impact the chapter holds in relation to job responsibilities and functions.

The first step in a communication plan is to include aspects of this chapter in the job application form and credentials application. Those applying for jobs and physician privileges need not apply if they are not willing to adhere to and respect patients' rights. For example, you could include the following language in your application:

> *By signing this application, I agree to treat patients and families with respect, ensure the patient's privacy and confidentiality of health information, and to review the patient's rights and responsibility notice.*

2.2 Chapter Captain Checklist for the Rights and Responsibilities of the Individual (RI) Chapter

Tasks	Completed (Date)	Not Completed (Date to Complete)
Review chapter		
Select team		
Review chapter with team		
Assign tasks to team: (Suggested quarterly and monthly closer to survey time frame) • Tracers • Chart reviews • Document reviews • Other		
Conduct PPR and identify areas of noncompliance and develop action plans for resolution. (Team can be involved as needed.)		
Provide educational opportunities for all staff related to chapter (e.g., newsletters, face-to-face, intranet tips for compliance, posters, Joint Commission fair)		
Stay abreast of any changes in standards and EPs for chapter		
Ask the following questions about documents: 1. Is the patient handbook up-to-date with regard to the RI chapter? 2. Is all posted signage available in another language? 3. Are patient rights and responsibilities signs posted and in another language? 4. Are all applicable forms (e.g., informed consents) up-to-date, available in another language, and at the appropriate level of understanding? 5. Are all applicable policies up-to-date?		

Note: This list can be added to as needed.

Communication regarding patients' rights should always be part of orientation to new board members, physicians, and staff. Some hospitals require all three groups to sign a document attesting that they will abide by and uphold these rights.

Ongoing communication is important for compliance with the patient rights chapter. In particular, the following topics should be considered for educational sessions or communication reminders:

- Respecting cultural and personal values, beliefs, and preferences
- Privacy and confidentiality
- Understanding how patients understand (i.e., health literacy)
- Advance directives and end-of-life decisions
- Informed consent
- Research/clinical trials
- Dealing with disruptive people (e.g., physicians, staff, patients, family members)
- Identifying neglect, exploitation, and verbal, mental, physical, and sexual abuse
- Resolving patient complaints

Communicating With Patients

Many of the topics previously mentioned can be incorporated into community educational programs for patients as well. However, at any point of entry to the hospital, whether inpatient or outpatient, the patient should be provided an outline of his or her rights and responsibilities. Part 3 will provide some ideas on how best to communicate this with patients.

Communicating With the Survey Team

A crucial role of the chapter captain and the members of this team is to educate staff and others with regard to questions the surveyors may ask during the survey. The surveyors will be observing, reviewing medical records, and talking to patients during the on-site survey. Being well-prepared to respond to surveyors' questions about patient rights is an essential part of a successful survey. Here are some questions that the rights chapter captain can prep staff with regard to compliance with this chapter:

Board

1. How are you educated with regard to patients' rights and responsibilities?

2. Do you have to sign a confidentiality statement with regard to patient information when you become a member of the board?

Physicians

1. How do you protect the patient's privacy during a bedside procedure?

2. Tell me about the process for informed consent to surgery.

3. Are the emergency department physicians educated with regard to the Emergency Medical Treatment and Active Labor Act (EMTALA)?

4. Do you honor a patient's advance directive?

Nursing and other clinical staff

1. Do you encourage patients to ask questions about their care and treatment?

2. Is there a chaplaincy program in the hospital?

3. What kind of educational tools do you use for patients who are blind?

4. How do you provide interpreters for patients who do not speak English?

5. How does a patient make a complaint about his or her care?

Registration staff

1. Do you provide all patients with the patient handbook?

2. Do you explain the rights and responsibilities to patients at the time of registration?

3. Do you explain the financial obligations of the patient?

HIM staff

1. How does someone obtain a copy of his or her medical record?

2. Who has access to the HIM department if it is closed?

3. Do you have to sign a confidentiality statement when you are hired?

In addition to questions, the surveyors will be observing the privacy of patients, especially in waiting areas, outside procedure rooms, and in the emergency department. Other observations focus on medical records, white boards, and computer screens that are not secure or in areas viewable by the public. Signage—for example, EMTALA—should be posted in other languages.

The previous information will work well as the rights team conducts mock tracers and educates staff for continuous survey readiness!

The Impact of the Patient Rights Chapter

The impact of the patient rights chapter is far reaching to the caregiver, nurses, staff, physicians, and patients because it gives them the tools necessary to properly communicate patient rights and responsibilities to all parties to ensure continual survey readiness.

First and foremost, then, the patient will feel respected, empowered, and confident that his or her wishes will be carried out. Caregivers, nurses, and staff will understand their respective roles and work toward developing a sense of trust between themselves and their patients.

Physicians will be obligated to respect their patients' wishes and will involve them in care decisions along with keeping their patients better informed of what is going on with their treatment. Physicians will have to be willing to round daily on patients, to regularly document in the medical record, and to adhere to policies that outline the requirements related to patients' rights.

PART 3

Implementing Patient Rights

This section will provide suggestions for implementing the patient rights chapter and how to maintain compliance. Although all chapters are important for proper implementation and continued compliance, the patient rights chapter is so focused on the patients' rights and responsibilities that a slip in noncompliance can present problems that can have a far-reaching impact on the patient, the reputation of the hospital, and can even result in legal issues.

However, it is a chapter that is straightforward and unambiguous, so compliance should be easy. At the end of this book, you will have the information and tools to sustain compliance, educate staff, and be ready for a survey at any time.

Designing and Implementing Policies

Let's start with policies! The patient rights chapter is clear in its requirements to have policies for selected elements of performance and to have these policies are implemented. As you review the chapter, policies and/or documentation requirements are designated by a "D" in a circle. The following are the required policies set forth in the chapter:

- General policy on patients' rights
- Informed consent
- Advance directives, withdrawing life-sustaining treatment, and withholding resuscitative services
- Organ donation
- Complaints
- Patient responsibilities
- Policy that addresses situations in which patients work for or on behalf of the hospital (for psychiatric hospital settings)

Figure 3.1 and Figure 3.2 give sample policies for rights and responsibilities of the individual and communication barriers, respectively. These sample policies can be used as a template to create other policies.

3.1 Sample Patients' Rights and Responsibilities Policy

Policy Name:	Patients' Rights and Responsibilities
Policy No:	1
Written by:	
Approved by:	
Origin Date:	
Revision Date(s):	
Purpose:	To define the patients' rights and responsibilities with regard to care, treatment, and services

Policy:

Each patient receiving care, treatment, and services is entitled to the rights as outlined in this policy. Each patient will be informed of his or her rights at the time of registration for care, treatment, and services.

The patient also has responsibilities as outlined in this policy and will be informed of them at the time of registration for care, treatment, and services.

Patients have the right to:

- Be treated in a dignified and respectful manner
- Communication in an effective manner that meets his or her needs
- Respect for cultural and personal values, beliefs, and preference
- Privacy
- Pain management
- Religious and other spiritual services
- Have a family member, friend, or others present for emotional support (this person may or may not be the patient's surrogate decision-maker or legally authorized representative)
- Not be discriminated against based on age, race, ethnicity, religion, culture, language, physical or mental disability, socioeconomic status, sex, sexual orientation, or gender identity or expression
- Have their primary care doctor notified when admitted or treated

3.1 Sample Patients' Rights and Responsibilities Policy *(cont.)*

Patients are responsible for:

- Providing information that assists in their care, treatment, and services
- Asking questions and acknowledging when they do not understand their care, treatment, and services
- Following instructions, policies, rules, and regulations to promote a safe environment and promote quality care practices
- Conducting themselves in a civil manner
- Meeting their financial responsibilities

References:

Joint Commission Accreditation Manual for Hospitals

Rights and Responsibilities of the Individual

RI.01.01.01, EP 1; RI.02.01.01, EP 1

Federal

State

Other related policies might include release of information, confidentiality and security of medical records, amendments to the medical record, research and clinical trials, abuse and neglect, healthcare literacy, nondiscrimination, use of a surrogate decision maker, and those contained in Appendix B. The medical staff bylaws, rules, and regulations and/or policies can also address some of these topics; in particular, informed consent, advance directives, withdrawing life-sustaining treatment, and withholding resuscitative services.

3.2 Sample Communication Barriers Policy

Policy Name:	Communication Barriers
Policy No:	2
Written by:	
Approved by:	
Origin Date:	
Revision Date(s):	
Purpose:	To provide assistance to all patients with communication barriers.

Policy:

Each patient with barriers to communication will receive the appropriate resource to understand and participate in his or her care, treatment, and services provided by the hospital. This includes foreign language, hearing, sight, speech, and mental barriers. These services are provided free of charge.

Services can be arranged and provided for by contacting your nurse manager, the case management department, or the nursing supervisor.

- Foreign language interpreters
- Hearing impaired
- Blind
- Mental barriers

Provide specific hospital detail under each heading. This information is also included in the patient handbook.

References:

Joint Commission Accreditation Manual for Hospitals

Rights and Responsibilities of the Individual

RI.01.01.03, EPs 1, 2, and 3

Federal

State

A regular review of policies—at least once a year—compared against the standards will ensure policies are accurate and up-to-date with current requirements. Policies should be reviewed for the following:

- Changes needed with regard to revised standards and elements of performance since the last review
- Proper templates used as required by the hospital
- Revision dates on the policy
- New policies that might be needed
- Education of staff
- Old policies are removed from source site; new policies posted

The Patient Handbook

Most hospitals provide the patient with a handbook upon admission or outpatient treatment that provides information helpful to the patient and family during a hospitalization or treatment. This is the ideal place to outline the patients' rights and responsibilities; use the chapter as a guide for sections and/or topics to include in the handbook. At the time of registration, pertinent sections related to the chapter should be pointed out by staff to the patient and/or family. Because the admission process can often be confusing to patients, some organizations place handbooks in patients' rooms and have the patients' rights and responsibilities posted on the television sets in patients' rooms and waiting areas.

Generally, a patient handbook will include the following:

- Welcome from the senior leader
- Mission and vision statements
- Patients' rights and responsibilities
- Notice of privacy practices
- How to contact The Joint Commission and other regulatory bodies
- How to make a complaint
- Visiting hours
- Access to health literacy needs (e.g., interpreters)
- Financial responsibilities:
  - Obtaining medical records
  - Chaplaincy program
  - Advance directives

The rights chapter captain and team can spearhead development and/or an annual review of the patient handbook because many of the topics to be covered are included in the patient rights chapter.

The Medical Staff

Often, medical staff can be a challenge when it comes to education and sustaining adherence to the patient rights chapter. Physicians are busy taking care of patients and are not always tuned in to the details outlined in standards and elements of performance. Frequent reminders of physician responsibilities in informing patients, such as helping them to understand and exercise their rights and treatment modalities and options; respecting their values, beliefs and preferences; and facilitating end-of-life decisions will help reduce the challenges facing those responsible for educating the medical staff.

Regular presentations to the medical executive committee and department meetings by the chapter captain or accreditation director will go a long way at reinforcing the medical staff's responsibility with regard to this chapter. Posters and messages on physician portals can also be used to sustain compliance.

An example of a presentation to the medical executive committee could cover the following points:

- Requirements of the rights and responsibilities of the individual chapter
- Examples of how the hospital meets the standards
- Examples from the medical staff bylaws, rules, and regulations that cover the standards (e.g., informed consent, advance directives)
- Examples of how the medical staff leaders support the standards (e.g., dealing with physician who do not show respect to their patients)

Other Caregivers, Nurses, and Staff

Maintaining compliance and ownership with other caregivers, nurses, and staff should be a simple task of providing updates at department meetings, conducting tracers, and providing some reminders through electronic communications, newsletters, and posters with tips and tools for compliance.

An annual Joint Commission "fun" fair is another way to sustain compliance and to provide continuing education with a special booth and prizes for this chapter. Consider also a Joint Commission intranet website that provides information related to the standards, tracer tools, and other resources for compliance.

The Board and Senior Leadership

Do not forget the board and senior leadership because they have to set the tone for respectful treatment of patients. Put the patient rights chapter on the agenda at least once a year and provide an overview at board and senior leadership meetings.

Tracers and Chart Reviews

There are no better ways to ensure compliance and understanding of this chapter than through patient tracers and chart reviews. Tracers and chart reviews get the team out on the units and in the departments making observations with regard to signage, privacy and confidentiality, and interviewing staff, to mention a few. Chart reviews ensure that necessary documentation is in the record (e.g., evidence of informed consent, advance directives, language barriers, learning needs). The team cannot just go through the chapter and make a guess that a policy is "somewhere" or a sign is printed in another language. They need to go see for themselves and, along the way, interview and educate staff to the standards and importance of the regulations.

The chapter leader should develop an annual schedule for tracers that will focus on this chapter, which includes the tool to be used and who will conduct the tracers. At least quarterly, a focused patients' rights tracer should be carried out. Aspects of the chapter can be incorporated into other tracers as well.

Figure 3.3 provides a sample calendar outlining the tasks to be done monthly, quarterly, and annually.

Requirements of this chapter, such as documentation of advance directives, pain management, informed consent, withholding life support, and clinical trials and research can be included as part of ongoing chart reviews. The grid in Part 1 can easily be adapted to tracer and ongoing chart review tools, like the one given in Figure 3.4.

3.3 Chapter Leader Calendar

Monthly	Quarterly	Annually
1. Facilitate monthly team meetings. 2. Conduct patient tracers. 3. Monitor and resolve outstanding issues. 4. Provide education. 5. Provide status report to accreditation director.	1. Publish newsletter. 2. Provide status report to senior leaders. 3. Provide status report to medical staff leadership. 4. Collect required documents for survey.	1. Complete annual PPR and identify noncompliance issues. 2. Develop action plan to resolve noncompliance issues. 3. Determine if team membership needs changes. 4. Educate new team members. 5. Establish and publish team meeting schedule. 6. Develop mock survey schedule. 7. Develop education plan.

3.4 Rights and Responsibilities of the Individual (RI) Tracer Tool

Standard and Element of Performance	Compliant	Not Compliant	Evidence of Standard Compliance or Action Steps If Not Compliant
RI.01.01.01 Respects, protects, and promotes patient rights			
EP1 Written policies			
EP2 Informing the patient of rights and responsibilities			
EP4 Treating the patient with dignity and respect			
EP5 Effective communication			
EP6 Respecting cultural and personal values, beliefs, preferences			
EP7 Rights to privacy			
EP8 Pain management			
EP9 Religious and other spiritual services			
RI.01.01.03 Receiving information in a way the patient understands			
EP1 Tailored to age, language, and ability to understand			
EP2 Providing interpreting and translation services			
EP3 Communicating effectively with regards to vision, speech, hearing, or cognitive impairments			
RI.01.02.01 Rights to participate in decisions regarding care, treatment, and services			
EP1 Notifying physician immediately			
EP2 Written information about the right to refuse care			
EP3 Right to refuse care in writing to the patient			
EP6 Rights for a surrogate decision-maker when patient is unable to make decisions			
EP7 Rights of the surrogate decision-maker is respected			
EP8 Involvement of the family in care decisions to the extent permitted by patient or surrogate decision-maker			

3.4 Rights and Responsibilities of the Individual (RI) Tracer Tool *(cont.)*

Standard and Element of Performance	Compliant	Not Compliant	Evidence of Standard Compliance or Action Steps If Not Compliant
EP20 Patient and surrogate decision-maker provided with information about the outcomes of care			
EP21 Patient and surrogate decision-maker provided information about unanticipated outcomes of care that relate to TJC identified sentinel events			
EP22 Licensed, independent practitioner responsible for the care informs the patient of unanticipated outcomes of care			
RI.01.03.01 Right to give or withhold informed consent			
EP1 Required policy outlines			
EP2 Care, treatment, and services that require informed consent			
EP3 Exceptions to informed consent			
EP4 Process to obtain informed consent			
EP5 Documentation in the medical record			
EP6 When a surrogate decision-maker may give consent			
EP7 Content related to proposed care, treatment, and services			
EP9 Benefits, risks, side effects, achieving goals, problems with recuperation			
EP11 Alternatives			
EP12 When information must be discussed or disclosed			
EP13 Emergency situations			
RI.0103.03 Give or withhold informed consent to produce or use recordings, films, other images for purposes other than care			
EP1 Obtains informed consent from patient for use other than care			

3.4 Rights and Responsibilities of the Individual (RI) Tracer Tool *(cont.)*

EP2 Documentation of informed consent and recordings, etc., are to be used			
EP3 Inability to obtain consent, production may occur if according to policy established through ethical mechanism			
EP4 Product remains in hospital's possession until patient's permission is obtained			
EP5 If consent not obtained, production is destroyed, or nonconsenting patient is removed from production			
EP6 Patient is informed of right to request cessation of production			
EP7 Confidential statement signed by any not bound by hospital policy			
EP8 Patient can rescind consent			
RI.01.03.05 Research, investigation, and clinical trials			
EP1 Hospital reviews all research protocols and weighs risks and benefits			
EP2 Information provided to patient (e.g., purpose, duration, description, benefits, risks, discomforts and side effects, advantageous alternative care)			
EP3 Refusal will not jeopardize care			
EP4 Research consent form documents information to make decision to participate			
EP5 Patient informed that refusal has no bearing on care			
EP6 Name of person providing information and date form is signed			
EP7 Consent describes patient's rights to privacy, confidentiality, and safety			
EP9 All information given to patient is kept in medical record			

3.4 Rights and Responsibilities of the Individual (RI) Tracer Tool *(cont.)*

Standard and Element of Performance	Compliant	Not Compliant	Evidence of Standard Compliance or Action Steps If Not Compliant
RI.01.04.01 Patient's right to receive information about the person responsible for care and those providing care			
EP1 Patient is informed of the name of the physician, clinical psychologist, or other practitioner primarily responsible for care			
EP2 Patient is informed of the name of the physician, clinical psychologist or other practitioner providing care			
RI.01.05.01 End-of-life decisions			
EP1 Written policies related to advance directives, forgoing or withdrawing life-sustaining treatment, and withholding resuscitative services			
EP4 Define if advance directive will be honored for outpatient services			
EP5 Advance directives are implemented			
EP6 Patient provided with written information about advance directives, withdrawing life-sustaining treatment, and withholding resuscitative services			
EP8 On admission, patient provided with information on extent hospital is able, unable, or unwilling to honor and advance directive			
EP9 Documents whether patient does or does not have advance directives			
EP10 Provides assistance if patient wishes to formulate an advance directive			
EP11 Those involved in care are aware of whether patient has an advance directive			
EP12 Patient's right to formulate, review, or revise advance directive is honored			

3.4 Rights and Responsibilities of the Individual (RI) Tracer Tool *(cont.)*

EP13 Hospital honors advance directives according to law, regulations, and hospital capabilities			
EP15 Documentation regarding patient's wishes concerning organ donation			
EP16 Hospital honors patient's wishes concerning organ donation			
EP17 Existence or lack of advance directive does not determine patient's right to access care			
EP19 In outpatient settings, policy on advance directives is communicated to patients			
EP20 In outpatient settings, patients are referred to resources for assistance with formulating advance directive			
EP21 Deemed status only: How permission to obtained and documented is defined			
RI.01.06.03 Patient is free from neglect; exploitation; and verbal, mental physical, and sexual abuse			
EP1 Hospital determines how patients will be protected from neglect, exploitation, and abuse during care			
EP2 All allegations, observations, and suspected cases of neglect, exploitation, and abuse are investigated			
EP3 All of the above are reported to authorities based on evaluations			
RI.01.06.05 Environment preserves dignity and contributes to a positive self-image			
EP2 Hospital settings providing longer term care (> 30 days) consider the number of patients assigned to a room (e.g., age, developmental levels, clinical conditions, diagnosis needs, hospital goals)			
EP4 Use of personal possessions and clothing			
EP15 Offers telephone and mail service			
EP16 Offers access to private telephones if patient requests			

3.4 Rights and Responsibilities of the Individual (RI) Tracer Tool *(cont.)*

Standard and Element of Performance	Compliant	Not Compliant	Evidence of Standard Compliance or Action Steps If Not Compliant
EP17 Restricting visitors, mail, telephone calls, or other forms of communication must be made with the participation and family, if appropriate			
EP18 Any restrictions as noted in EP17 must be documented in the medical record			
EP19 Any restrictions as noted in EPs 17 and 18 must be evaluated for therapeutic effectiveness			
RI.01.07.01 Patient and family complaints must be reviewed			
EP1 Complaint resolution process is established			
EP2 Patient and family are informed about the process			
EP4 Hospital resolves complaints if possible			
EP6 Patient is notified when complaint cannot be resolved immediately and follows up			
EP7 Phone number and address needed to file a complaint with state authority are provided to the patient			
EP10 Patient has right to voice complaints and recommend changes freely			
EP18 Deemed status – Patient is provided a written notice of decisions related to complaints to include name of hospital contact person, steps taken in investigation, results, date completed process			
EP19 Deemed status – Time frames are established for review and response			
EP20 Deemed status – Process for resolving complaints includes a timely referral of patient concerns about quality of care and premature discharges to the quality improvement organization (QIO)			

3.4 Rights and Responsibilities of the Individual (RI) Tracer Tool *(cont.)*

RI.01.07.03 – Rights to protective and advocacy services			
EP1 Patients needing protective services are provided resources to family and the courts			
EP2 List of names, addresses, and telephone numbers of advocacy groups is maintained			
EP3 Advocacy list given to patient when requested			
RI.01.07.07 – For psychiatric hospital settings with stays over 30 days, patients rights are protected if they work for or on behalf of the hospital			
EP1 Written policy			
EP2 Policy is implemented			
EP3 Wages paid to patients are in accordance with law and regulations			
EP4 Work performed by the patient is incorporated into the plan of care			
EP5 Patients have the right to refuse work			
RI.02.01.01 Patient responsibilities			
EP1 Written policy			
EP2 Hospital informs patient about his or her responsibilities			

NOTE: Each EP can be turned into a question while conducting tracers. You can make observations, ask staff questions, and review documents.

Impact on Patient Care

In closing, the impact of this chapter on patient care cannot be minimized. When the requirements of this chapter are implemented and embraced by the leaders, the healthcare team, and the patient, the quality of patient care and safety will rise exponentially.

As previously stated at the beginning of this book, it is only when patients understand their illness and what types of care, treatments, and services can be provided will they be able to make good decisions about their care. It is the responsibility of the hospital to provide an atmosphere of respect and open communication with patients from the minute they present for care and treatment. It is everyone's job to encourage patient participation by informing them of their rights, providing avenues for participation in their care, and establishing a partnership between the patient and the caregivers.

The more caregivers know about the patient, the better the care decisions will be. And, in many cases, the patient will recover faster and follow instructions once he or she is at home. It just makes sense: The more you know, the better the care, resulting in a more compliant patient in following instructions to full recovery.

APPENDIX A

Rights and Responsibilities of the Individual (RI) Checklist

The standards in the RI chapter set forth a framework to ensure that the processes supporting patient rights, proper consideration of patients and their families, cultural sensitivity, and communication with patients and families are sound.

The use of practice tracers makes it easy to gauge performance in some of the key requirements, such as:

- The process(es) in place to identify and address advance directives
- Use of appropriate assists to ensure clear communication with patients and significant others, such as interpreter services
- Implementation of a credible informed consent process
- Identification of and intervention on behalf of potential victims of abuse

The RI concepts support the culture of safety that surveyors expect to find throughout your organization (see Leadership chapter). They also respond to increasing consumer expectation for transparency in our communication with patients and families. This is definitely an area where great policies are not sufficient. It's not enough to "talk the talk"; this is an area where all of your staff is expected to "walk the talk"!

*All content and figures contained in Appendix A are taken from *The Joint Commission Mock Tracer Made Simple.* Published by HCPro, Inc.

REQUIREMENT D P	RI.01.01.01 Respect for Patients' Rights			
Elements of Compliance	**Yes**	**No**	**Sometimes**	**Examples of Compliance**
1. Do you have policies and procedures that address patients' rights to care, treatment, and services within your organization's scope and in compliance with state and federal laws/regulations?	☐	☐	☐	Organizationwide policies clearly require access to services by all seeking services provided by the organization, specific protections while a patient, and a safe process for transfer or referral when patients' needs are outside the organization's mission and scope.
2. Do you provide all patients with information about their rights?	☐	☐	☐	A brochure on patient rights and responsibilities is provided to each patient at the time of registration. In addition, these brochures are posted in patient rooms and available in patient waiting rooms throughout the organization.
3. Do all staff demonstrate respect for the personal dignity of each patient?	☐	☐	☐	Staff members demonstrate respect for patients by calling them Ms., Mr., Mrs., with surname, drawing cubicle curtains, treating their personal belongings with respect, etc.
4. Do staff respect the patients' right to clear, easily understood communication?	☐	☐	☐	Staff demonstrate this by using appropriate educational materials, obtaining interpreter services, or obtaining TTY devices for hearing-impaired patients.
5. Do staff members understand that patients' cultural, spiritual, psychosocial, and personal values, beliefs, and preferences must be respected to extent permissible under law?	☐	☐	☐	New employee orientation includes a section on respect for each patient's beliefs. This is reinforced in departmental orientation in relation to job-specific issues that may arise.
6. Do staff demonstrate respect for patient privacy?	☐	☐	☐	Staff demonstrate respect for privacy by drawing cubicle curtains, discussing confidential information in private, closing exam room doors, providing robes for gowned patients, knocking before entering a room, etc.
7. Does your organization have mechanisms in place to support the patient's right to have his or her pain managed, to the extent possible, including:				Our organization's approach to pain management starts with assessment of all patients regarding the presence, intensity, location, character, and methods of relief of pain. All clinical staff have been educated regarding the importance of pain management and the need to reassess for effectiveness of interventions. Educational materials are provided to patients and families to explain the steps they can take to partner in pain management.
• Assessment?	☐	☐	☐	
• Education for clinical staff?	☐	☐	☐	
• Education for patients/families?	☐	☐	☐	
• Reassessment?	☐	☐	☐	

REQUIREMENT D P	RI.01.01.01 Respect for Patients' Rights (cont.)			
Elements of Compliance	**Yes**	**No**	**Sometimes**	**Examples of Compliance**
8. Is there a process in place to access spiritual and pastoral services when requested?	☐	☐	☐	Each patient is asked about spiritual/pastoral needs during initial assessment. A consult is made if the patient desires a visit. Special effort is made at the time of patient/family crisis.
9. Does the patient receive specific information addressing the right to access, request changes to, or receive an accounting of disclosures regarding his or her health information?	☐	☐	☐	The brochure on patient rights and responsibilities clearly describes the patient's right to access, amend, or receive an accounting of disclosure of personal healthcare information. The privacy officer's phone number is included for questions in this matter.

WHAT YOUR POLICY SHOULD INCLUDE: **POLICY NO:** ______________ **POLICY LOCATION:** ______________

An organizationwide policy listing all patient rights should exist. It's common to include patient responsibilities in the same policy. Specific procedures, such as the mechanism to access pastoral services or the process for stabilization and transfer of patients who need services that you do not provide, serve to operationalize your organization's approach to patient rights. Policy should clearly state the need to provide information on rights and responsibilities to each patient. Note: Be sure to check state and federal regulations regarding patient rights when drafting or revising this policy.

REQUIREMENT	RI.01.01.03 Effective Communication			
Elements of Compliance	**Yes**	**No**	**Sometimes**	**Examples of Compliance**
1. Are written materials, such as brochures, forms, and instructions, in language that can be understood?	☐	☐	☐	Written materials for adults are at sixth-grade reading level; most frequently used forms and instructions have been translated into the top three languages.
2. Are interpretive services available?	☐	☐	☐	Interpretive services for top three non-English languages are available on-site 24/7. Other languages are provided through via on-call service or language line service.
3. Are mechanisms available for communicating with those with hearing, vision, speech, language, and cognitive deficits?	☐	☐	☐	Staff members have been trained in the appropriate methods of communicating with patients with physical or cognitive barriers.

WHAT YOUR POLICY SHOULD INCLUDE: POLICY NO: ______________ POLICY LOCATION: ______________

None specifically required by the standards; however, check state and federal requirements, especially related to interpreter services.

REQUIREMENT	RI.01.02.01 Involving Patients in Care Decisions Formulary			
Elements of Compliance	**Yes**	**No**	**Sometimes**	**Examples of Compliance**
1. Are all patients involved in decisions about their care and treatment options?	☐	☐	☐	Members of the healthcare team involve patients in discussions about the plan of care and treatment, including discharge planning. When DNR orders are suspended for a procedure, there is a discussion with the patient/decision-maker regarding the implications, and the discussion is documented in the progress notes.
2. To the extent possible, are all patients involved in resolving questions about care and treatment?	☐	☐	☐	
3. Do patients receive written information about the right to refuse treatment, including end-of-life treatment?	☐	☐	☐	
4. Are your patients informed of their right to refuse care/treatment, to the extent allowed by law?	☐	☐	☐	When questions regarding care and treatment arise, the patient is involved in discussions about "next steps" and alternatives. (See also RI.01.03.01, Informed Consent.)
5. Is it your practice to identify and work with a surrogate decision-maker when the patient is unable to speak for himself or herself?	☐	☐	☐	The brochure on patient rights and responsibilities outlines the right to refuse treatment, including resuscitation, when death is imminent.
6. Do staff show respect for the legally responsible representative's responsibility to make care decisions, including the right to refuse care?	☐	☐	☐	The brochure on patient rights and responsibilities clearly identifies the patient's or the surrogate decision-maker's right to refuse care/treatment within the law. Special issues regarding refusal of treatment for minors, parents with minor children, and pregnant women are referred to the ethics committee or legal counsel.
7. Is the family, according to the patient's wishes and according to law, involved in decisions about care and treatment?	☐	☐	☐	
8. Do you inform patients/surrogate decision-makers and families, as appropriate, about outcomes of care, treatment, and services to provide them with the facts they need to participate in future care decisions?	☐	☐	☐	Guidelines exist to determine the appropriate decision-maker when the patient is a minor or unable to speak for himself or herself. Legal guardians, healthcare proxies, or family members (according to next-of-kin hierarchy) are identified; the name of this person(s) is documented in the medical record.
9. Do you inform patients/surrogate decision-makers and families, as appropriate, about unexpected outcomes that are the result of a sentinel event, when the patient is not already aware or when there is a need for dialogue?	☐	☐	☐	A review of medical records demonstrates that the legally responsible representative approves decisions when the patient is unable to do so. The family is involved in decision-making with the patient's permission as appropriate.
10. Is the responsible LIP or designee the person who discloses unexpected outcomes with the patient and family as appropriate?	☐	☐	☐	The practice of informing patients of outcomes of care, treatment, or services, whether positive or negative, is understood in our organization. When significant unexpected outcomes as a result of a sentinel event must be disclosed, the risk manager is available to assist the physician or designee in

REQUIREMENT	RI.01.02.01 Involving Patients in Care Decisions Formulary (cont.)	
Elements of Compliance	**Yes No Sometimes**	**Examples of Compliance**
		doing so. The investigation of a sentinel event includes a check to be sure that the patient/family have been informed and that all their questions have been addressed. The discussion with the patient/family is documented in a brief progress note.

WHAT YOUR POLICY SHOULD INCLUDE: POLICY NO: ______________ POLICY LOCATION: ______________

A policy is not specifically required by standard. Development of guidelines is recommended for both substituted judgment and disclosure of unanticipated outcomes.

REQUIREMENT D P **RI.01.03.01 Informed Consent**

Elements of Compliance	Yes	No	Sometimes	Examples of Compliance
1. Do you have a policy (or policies) addressing informed consent (IC)? Does it:				An organizationwide policy on IC defines the categories of procedures, treatments, care, and services that carry significant risk and therefore require IC. The physician is responsible for IC and is required to use approved forms, which are filed in the medical record once completed. Policy prohibits performing the procedure/treatment without IC except in an emergency, the nature of which must be documented in the medical record. There are guidelines to determine the appropriate decision-maker when the patient is incompetent, unconscious, or a minor.
• Identify treatments and procedures that require IC?	☐	☐	☐	
• Identify situations when normally required IC can be omitted, such as in an extreme emergency?	☐	☐	☐	
• Detail the steps to follow to obtain IC?	☐	☐	☐	
• Describe the format for documenting IC in the record?	☐	☐	☐	
• Provide guidelines for involvement of a surrogate decision-maker in instances when the patient is unable to give IC?	☐	☐	☐	
2. Does your IC process incorporate discussion of all required elements of IC—specifically, the:				IC forms are completed in full, according to policy, and filed in the legal section of the medical record. The forms are designed to meet Joint Commission as well as any state or federal requirements.
• Description of proposed procedures, treatments, etc.?	☐	☐	☐	
• Risks, benefits, known side effects, or post-treatment/post procedure issues?	☐	☐	☐	A review of medical records for procedures, treatment, or services requiring IC demonstrates the level of compliance with the policy.
• Likelihood of reaching the desired outcome?	☐	☐	☐	
• Alternatives and risks/benefits, side effects of these, including the alternative of doing nothing?	☐	☐	☐	
• Limitations on protecting the confidentiality of patient information?	☐	☐	☐	
3. Is the IC policy followed consistently?	☐	☐	☐	

WHAT YOUR POLICY SHOULD INCLUDE: **POLICY NO:** ____________ **POLICY LOCATION:** ____________

An organizationwide policy that defines when informed consent is required, the process for obtaining and documenting it, role of surrogates, the right of the patient to refuse consent, and how the process is monitored. It clearly states that the procedure/treatment will not commence until consent is obtained, except in an emergency. Be sure to include all state and federal requirements. Any forms approved for use are attached to the policy.

REQUIREMENT D P **RI.01.03.03 Consent for Filming or Recording**

Elements of Compliance	Yes	No	Sometimes	Examples of Compliance
1. Do you obtain informed consent for visual or audio recording for nonclinical use inside your organization as part of your general consent for treatment?	☐	☐	☐	The organization's standard informed consent include a clause stipulating that filming or recording may be performed for use in-house for orientation purposes and educational programs.
2. Do you obtain specific, written informed consent for visual or audio recording that will be used outside your organization?	☐	☐	☐	When taping or recording of a patient is performed for viewing outside the organization, such as marketing videos or training films for use at the local community college, specific consent is obtained prior to initiation.
3. Do you obtain the above consent prior to filming or recording (except in special circumstances outlined below)?	☐	☐	☐	
4. If the patient is unable to consent prior to filming or recording, do you have a policy that addresses ethical concerns to guide staff in this situation?	☐	☐	☐	An organizationwide policy, developed and approved through the Ethics Committee, describes the limitations on filming or recording of patients who are unable to grant consent; for instance, filming or recording performed as part of a diagnostic procedure may be done, but filming or recording for use in marketing materials is prohibited when consent is not obtained.
5. Is use of the resulting media delayed until informed consent is obtained?	☐	☐	☐	
6. In instances where the consent is never obtained, is the media destroyed or altered to delete inclusion of the non-consenting patient(s)?	☐	☐	☐	Patients are informed that the proceedings may be halted at any time.
7. Are patients informed of their right to request that filming or recording be stopped?	☐	☐	☐	It's standard practice to have all vendors with patient contact sign a business associate agreement.
8. If outside help is used in the filming or recording, are they required to sign confidentiality statements?	☐	☐	☐	

WHAT YOUR POLICY SHOULD INCLUDE: **POLICY NO:** __________ **POLICY LOCATION:** __________

An organizationwide policy describes the requirements for consent for visual and audio recording of patients. It differentiates between materials that will be used within the organization and materials that will be shared with those outside the organization. The overriding principle is protection of the patient's privacy and confidentiality. When patients cannot give their consent, special safeguards require that materials developed without consent are not used until consent is granted and that they are destroyed if consent is not obtained in a reasonable amount of time.

REQUIREMENT D	RI.01.03.05 Protection of Research Subjects			
Elements of Compliance	**Yes**	**No**	**Sometimes**	**Examples of Compliance**
1. Does your organization review each proposed research protocol to determine its fit with your mission, vision, and values, and also to gauge the relative benefit and risk to patients who might become subjects?	☐	☐	☐	An Institutional Review Board (IRB) is charged with the responsibility of receiving, reviewing, and approving/denying all requests to use a research protocol or investigational drug at our institution.
2. When research protocols are approved for use in your organization, do potential subjects receive ALL of the following information to guide their decision re: participation?				To give consent to participate in a research protocol, each potential subject must receive an explanation of the purpose; the proposed length of time for participation; a description of the risks, benefits, and side effects; any alternative therapies/treatments that might be beneficial; and a full description of the procedure that the patient will have to follow.
• Description of the purpose	☐	☐	☐	
• Length of time the patient will be involved	☐	☐	☐	
• Details on procedures the patient will be expected to follow	☐	☐	☐	
• Description of expected risks, benefits and reactions	☐	☐	☐	Every potential subject is informed that their decision to participate, or not participate, will not affect their access to other services of the organization.
• Any alternatives that might reasonably be provided in place of the research protocol	☐	☐	☐	
3. Are patients aware that their refusal to participate in a research protocol will not affect their access to other modes of care and treatment?	☐	☐	☐	The informed consent form for research protocols is designed to include all required information. The subject cannot be placed on the protocol until all fields are complete.
4. Is consent to participate in a research protocol documented on a form that includes:				All information provided to the research subject and the completed consent form are filed in a special section of the medical record.
• Adequate information about the project?	☐	☐	☐	
• A note that patient was informed that refusal will not interfere with access to any other services?	☐	☐	☐	
• The name of the person providing the information?	☐	☐	☐	
• Information about the patient's right to privacy, confidentiality, and safety?	☐	☐	☐	
• Any limitations to the confidentiality of the patient's personal identifiable private information?	☐	☐	☐	
• The date the form was signed?	☐	☐	☐	
5. Do you file a copy of all research information, provided in writing to the patient, in the medical record or a research file?	☐	☐	☐	

WHAT YOUR POLICY SHOULD INCLUDE: POLICY NO: ______________ POLICY LOCATION: ______________

Not required, but suggest that the IRB have written guidelines.

REQUIREMENT	RI.01.04.01 Patient Information Re: Physician			
Elements of Compliance	**Yes**	**No**	**Sometimes**	**Examples of Compliance**
1. Are patients informed of the name of the physician/practitioner responsible for their care and the name(s) of any physicians/practitioners performing care, treatment, or services?	☐	☐	☐	Physicians and other practitioners introduce themselves at their first interaction with patients and always wear photo IDs. When patients are admitted to the hospital in the care of a physician unknown to them, they receive written information in their admission packet and at discharge.

WHAT YOUR POLICY SHOULD INCLUDE: POLICY NO: ____________ POLICY LOCATION: ____________

Not applicable.

REQUIREMENT **RI.01.05.01 End-of-Life Issues**

Elements of Compliance	Yes	No	Sometimes	Examples of Compliance
1. Do you have written policies covering: • Advance directives? • Forgoing or removing life-sustaining treatment? • Withholding resuscitative services (DNR policy)?	 ☐ ☐ ☐	 ☐ ☐ ☐	 ☐ ☐ ☐	Organizationwide policies set forth the approach to end-of-life care and the decision-making regarding that care. Specific requirements regarding advance directives are addressed.
2. Does the policy on advance directives clearly state whether the hospital honors advance directives, and any limitations that might be imposed?	☐	☐	☐	Each inpatient is asked about existing advance directives, and to the extent that information is shared with the hospital, and within the limits of the law and hospital policy, all advance directives will be honored.
3. Does the policy address whether the hospital will honor advance directives in any outpatient settings?	☐	☐	☐	Ambulatory surgical and invasive procedure patients are asked for their advance directive status. The advance directive is honored in these settings when known. A review of medical records of patients who answer affirmatively to the advance directive inquiry reveals the compliance level for this requirement. Questions about advanced directives are included in practice tracers; documentation is monitored through ongoing medical record review.
4. Is the existence of an advance directive documented in the medical record?	☐	☐	☐	
5. Are advance directive policies implemented consistently?	☐	☐	☐	
6. Is a referral provided if a patient wishes to develop an advance directive?	☐	☐	☐	A social worker or patient representative will assist both inpatients and ambulatory patients in preparing advance directives.
7. Is there a mechanism in place to alert care providers to any existing advance directive?	☐	☐	☐	Advance directives are placed in the legal section of the record, and a sticker is placed on the cover to alert staff to the existence of an advance directive.
8. Is there evidence that staff understand the patient's right to review and change any existing advance directive?	☐	☐	☐	Every patient is advised of this right at the time that he or she creates an advance directive and reminded of it at the time of assessment.
9. Are patients' wishes regarding organ donation documented and honored, to the extent possible under the law and criteria for donation?	☐	☐	☐	The hospital has developed criteria, in concert with the OPO, to identify which deaths should be referred to the OPO. This is monitored through a death record review.
10. Do staff understand that advance directives, or lack thereof, have no bearing on access to services?	☐	☐	☐	Staff education has been provided regarding advance directives and the organization's responsibilities in this area.

WHAT YOUR POLICY SHOULD INCLUDE: **POLICY NO:** ______________ **POLICY LOCATION:** ______________

Organizationwide policies exist on advance directives, withdrawing or forgoing life-sustaining services, or withholding resuscitation services (DNR status). The advance directive policy clearly explains the process for ascertaining the presence of advance directives, the follow-up process for obtaining copies for the record, the mechanism for providing assistance in formulating directives, and the process for invoking the directive. Withdrawing or forgoing life-sustaining services is addressed in a policy that provides guidelines for a case-by-case review when considered. The DNR policy describes the type(s) of cases where this may be appropriate, the requirements for writing a DNR order, and the appropriate response by caregivers when a DNR order exists, or when a DNR order is suspended. Outpatient applicability is clearly stated in policy as appropriate. Respecting patient's wishes regarding organ or tissue donation is also addressed. Note: Faith-based hospitals need to specify any religious limitations to honoring advance directives.

REQUIREMENT D	RI.01.06.03 Freedom from Abuse and Neglect			
Elements of Compliance	**Yes**	**No**	**Sometimes**	**Examples of Compliance**
1. Does your organization take steps to prevent, to the best of your ability, abuse, neglect, and exploitation (real or perceived) of your patients by any party (staff, visitors, other patients, relatives)?	☐	☐	☐	All prospective employees are screened for criminal history. Employee orientation and annual education include information about the organization's stance on this issue, including action that will be taken against employees found to be responsible.
2. Do you promptly investigate any allegations of abuse, neglect, or exploitation?	☐	☐	☐	All possible instances of abuse, neglect, or exploitation are immediately investigated and appropriate action is taken, up to and including reporting to law enforcement authorities and state agencies.
3. Do you file reports to the proper authorities when your internal assessment of the suspected acts warrants it?	☐	☐	☐	

WHAT YOUR POLICY SHOULD INCLUDE:	POLICY NO: ______________ POLICY LOCATION: ______________
Not specifically required by the standard, but check your state regulations for requirements, including required postings.	

REQUIREMENT	RI.01.06.05 Preserving Dignity			
Elements of Compliance	**Yes**	**No**	**Sometimes**	**Examples of Compliance**
1. Are patient areas designed to help patients preserve their dignity and personal appearance?	☐	☐	☐	Patient rooms and waiting/change areas help to preserve a positive self-image and dignity. They are clean, are well-maintained, and have mirrors and space for grooming/proper hygiene.
Hospitals with LOS < 30 days:				
2. Is the number of patients in each room appropriate to the type of patients and the organization's goals?	☐	☐	☐	Accommodations for patients take into account patient age, safety factors, condition, services required, and diagnosis. The number of patients in each room may be kept below the maximum to address various factors.
3. Are patients allowed to keep personal items at the bedside, and even wear personal clothing, as appropriate to setting and patient's condition?	☐	☐	☐	Within the limits of clinical care and safety, patients are encouraged to wear personal clothing and continue their personal grooming habits while hospitalized.
4. Do you provide access to telephone, mail, or e-mail?	☐	☐	☐	
5. Do you provide privacy for telephone conversations? (Consider space and availability of telephones.)	☐	☐	☐	Patients are informed of the availability of private telephones for confidential conversations; wireless Internet access is available in most patient rooms and public spaces, and there is daily mail delivery.
Hospitals with LOS > 30 days:				
6. If a patient's access to communication with those outside the hospital must be limited, does the following occur?				On the adolescent behavioral unit, it is not unusual to have to limit the patient's access to the telephone during the course of therapy. When this is done, the patient is engaged in a discussion, along with parents/guardian, to detail the reasons for doing this and the specific behaviors that will be needed to regain telephone privileges. There is daily documentation in the record detailing the discussion and the patient's progress until the privileges are reinstated.
• The patient is involved in the decision	☐	☐	☐	
• There is a note placed in the record detailing the reasons for this limitation	☐	☐	☐	
• Limitations are evaluated for therapeutic effectiveness	☐	☐	☐	

WHAT YOUR POLICY SHOULD INCLUDE:	POLICY NO: ______________ POLICY LOCATION: ______________
Not applicable.	

REQUIREMENT	D RI.01.07.01 Resolving Complaints		
Elements of Compliance	**Yes No Sometimes**		**Examples of Compliance**
1. Is there a process for receiving, reviewing, and resolving complaints?	☐ ☐ ☐		There is an established process for receipt and review of all complaints. The hospital's patient advocates and the risk manager work together to ensure the process is followed. The patient rights and responsibilities brochure covers the process for resolving complaints as well as the right to make a complaint to the state department of public health or The Joint Commission. Phone numbers are provided for the organization's patient advocate, the DPH, and The Joint Commission. All significant complaints are addressed in writing; however, a face-to-face conference is always attempted as part of the resolution process. All medical staff members and employees know that complaints must never affect the patient's care or result in any type of coercion or retaliation.
2. Are patients informed about the process for resolution of complaints?	☐ ☐ ☐		
3. Do you respond to patients/families with complaints and attempt to resolve them, to the extent possible?	☐ ☐ ☐		
4. Do you have a formal process for addressing complaints that are significant (by hospital definition), including informing the patient/family of any follow-up action(s)?	☐ ☐ ☐		
5. Do you inform patients about their right to file a complaint with your state agency?	☐ ☐ ☐		
6. Are patients free to make complaints without fear of retaliation or impact to their care and treatment?	☐ ☐ ☐		

WHAT YOUR POLICY SHOULD INCLUDE: **POLICY NO:** __________ **POLICY LOCATION:** __________

Not specifically required by the standard, but suggest that a written process be put in place and that it address any applicable state or federal regulations regarding handling of complaints.

REQUIREMENT D	RI.01.07.03 Access to Protective Services	
Elements of Compliance	**Yes No Sometimes**	**Examples of Compliance**
1. Do you have mechanisms in place to identify patients who may benefit from protective services and to access the courts or other family services, to establish such services when needed?	☐ ☐ ☐	The assessment includes questions to help identify patients who may benefit from appointment of a guardian or provision of protective services (e.g., incompetent patients with no family, children at risk). Social workers are responsible for assessing the need and initiating steps to secure services, as appropriate.
2. Do you maintain a list of state and community client advocacy agencies to assist in this process?	☐ ☐ ☐	
3. Is this list available to patients upon request?	☐ ☐ ☐	A list of state and local advocacy services is maintained and updated periodically. This list is available for use by patients and families.

WHAT YOUR POLICY SHOULD INCLUDE: POLICY NO: __________ POLICY LOCATION: __________

Not applicable.

REQUIREMENT D P	RI.01.07.07 Patients Performing Work (Note: Applies only to hospitals with LOS > 30 days)			
Elements of Compliance	**Yes**	**No**	**Sometimes**	**Examples of Compliance**
1. Do policies and procedures define the circumstances in which patients may work at the hospital or perform duties that benefit the hospital?	☐	☐	☐	Departmental policy defines the circumstances under which a patient may engage in work for or on behalf of the hospital. The clinical indications, the type of work, the amount of time spent at work, and the pay associated with the assignment are all adequately addressed.
2. Are the policies and procedures followed by staff?	☐	☐	☐	A review of the cases where work was done shows the level of compliance with the policy.
3. Do the patients receive wages in compliance with law and regulation?	☐	☐	☐	The HR department sets the parameters for paying patients for work consistent with all laws and regulations.
4. Is the work assigned included in the plan for care and treatment?	☐	☐	☐	The work assignment and the expected therapeutic outcome are described in the plan of care. The work is reevaluated as part of the ongoing reassessment of the patient's progress.
5. Can the patient refuse to perform work?	☐	☐	☐	Patients may refuse work assignments. When this occurs, other activities are substituted with the goal of achieving the same therapeutic result.

WHAT YOUR POLICY SHOULD INCLUDE: **POLICY NO:** ______________ **POLICY LOCATION:** ______________

A policy and detailed procedure for engaging patients in work should include the clinical indications for presenting an opportunity to work; the types of work that can be offered; the number of hours per day, or per week, that a patient may be allowed to work; how the patient will be paid; how often the patient will be reassessed; how supervision will occur; any limitations that are applicable; and the patient's right to refuse the offer to work.

REQUIREMENT D P **RI.02.01.01 Patient Responsibilities**

Elements of Compliance	Yes	No	Sometimes	Examples of Compliance
1. Does your organization have a policy that defines the responsibilities of patients/families, which includes all of the following responsibilities?				An organizationwide policy identifies the brochure on patient rights and responsibilities as the mechanism for communicating responsibilities to patients and families.
• Sharing pertinent information	☐	☐	☐	The patient rights and responsibilities brochure advises patients to provide complete and accurate information to the best of their ability; requests them to ask questions whenever they don't understand, especially about their medications and treatments; explains why following instructions will help speed recovery; makes clear that they will have to accept the consequences of their own actions or inaction; sets expectations for following hospital policies such as visitor and smoking guidelines; and asks for their cooperation in showing respect for all and requests that they meet any obligations for payment.
• Asking questions	☐	☐	☐	
• Following directions and the agreed-upon care plan	☐	☐	☐	
• Accepting the consequences of their actions	☐	☐	☐	
• Following hospital policy and local/state regulations, as appropriate	☐	☐	☐	
• Demonstrating respect and consideration for hospital staff and fellow patients	☐	☐	☐	
• Fulfilling financial obligations	☐	☐	☐	
2. Do you inform patients of their responsibilities, either verbally or in writing, per hospital policy?	☐	☐	☐	The brochures are provided to all patients and are available throughout the organization in English, Spanish, Portuguese, and Haitian Creole.

WHAT YOUR POLICY SHOULD INCLUDE: **POLICY NO:** __________ **POLICY LOCATION:** __________

Usually covered in the policy on Patient Rights (RI.01.01.01), but may be separate if you so choose. Make sure all responsibilities in the standard are itemized.

APPENDIX B

Sample Policies and Procedures

It is imperative that the patient rights chapter have clear, effectively communicated policies for certain elements of performance.

Use the following sample policies on pain management, requests for information, advance directives, and patient complaints in your facility as templates to create other policies.

B.1 Sample Pain Management Policy

Policy name: Pain management
Policy number: 3
Written by:
Approved by:
Origin date:
Revision date(s):
Purpose: To respect the patient's right to pain management and be involved in decisions related to pain management

Policy:

All patients have the right to be involved in their pain management by expressing their pain in a manner that respects any communication barriers, to have relief from their pain, to be checked frequently to ensure pain relief, and to be involved in decisions regarding their pain.

Procedure:

1. Pain will be assessed initially upon admission to the hospital and in outpatient settings.
2. Pain will be assessed using a pain assessment tool that accommodates the patient's condition and ability to communicate.
3. The patient and family will be provided education regarding pain management.
4. Pain will be reassessed within ________ (hospital-specific time frame) of intervention, when new pain occurs, and upon changes in level of care.
5. Documentation of the initial assessment and reassessments will be entered into the medical record.
6. Pain will be based on a scale of 1 to 10, with 1–3 being mild, 4–7 moderate, and 8–10 severe.
7. The appropriate physicians will be notified and write orders for pain management, medications, and treatment.

References:

Joint Commission *Accreditation Manual for Hospitals*
Rights and Responsibilities of the Individual
RI.01.01.01, EP8

B.2 Sample Request for Information Policy

Policy name: Access, amendments, and disclosures of personal health information
Policy number: 4
Written by:
Approved by:
Origin date:
Revision date(s):
Purpose: To establish a policy and procedure for patients to access, request amendment to, and obtain information on disclosures of their personal health information

Policy:

All patients have the right to their personal health information, to obtain copies of their medical records, to request amendments to their medical records, and to receive full information on disclosures of their health information.

Procedure:

Obtaining copies of medical records:

1. The patient (or legal representative, based upon appropriate documented proof) presents to the health information management department (HIMD) with picture identification and signs the release of information form.
2. Unless an urgent medical need exists, the standard rate for copies will be applied.
3. Medical records may be provided in paper format or on a CD.
4. Records will not be released while the patient is hospitalized unless so ordered by the physician.
5. Other requests for medical records will be based upon signed authorization by the patient.

B.2 Sample Request for Information Policy *(cont.)*

Amendments to the medical records:

1. The patient presents to the HIMD with picture identification and completes the request to amend his or her medical record.
2. The patient is informed that changes to the original medical record cannot be made, but that his or her amendment will be entered into the medical record.
3. The physician of record will be notified.
4. An electronic file of all amendment requests will be maintained in the HIMD.

Disclosures of health information:

1. The patient presents to the HIMD with picture identification and completes the request for disclosure of his or her health information.
2. A copy of all disclosures will be provided to the patient in paper format or on CD.
3. The request will be filed in the medical record.

References:

Joint Commission *Accreditation Manual for Hospitals*

Rights and Responsibilities of the Individual

RI.01.01.01, EP8

B.3 Sample Advance Directives Policy

Policy name: Advance Directives
Policy number: 5
Written by:
Approved by:
Origin date:
Revision date(s):
Purpose: To identify patients with advance directives and to ensure that healthcare professionals and designated representatives honor the directives within state and federal laws; to provide patients with information related to advance directives; and to provide a process for patients to execute an advance directive

Policy:

Advance directives are generally identified as living wills or healthcare power of attorney, but each state should be queried to determine what constitutes a legal advance directive. _______________ identifies a legal advance directive as _______________________.

Procedure:

1. At the time of admission or outpatient registration, the registration staff will query the patient or legal representative as to the presence, absence, or interest in execution of an advance directive.
2. The information, based upon the patient's and/or legal representative's, will be entered into the appropriate area of the registration form.
3. If the patient or legal representative brings the advance directive to the hospital, a copy of the advance directive will become part of the legal medical record.
4. If the advance directive is not available at the time of registration, the registration staff will note this on the appropriate area of the registration form and request that a family member provide the advance directive as soon as possible to a member of the registration staff. The staff will enter the information into the appropriate area of the medical record and provide a copy for the medical record.

B.3 **Sample Advance Directives Policy *(cont.)***

5. The patient or legal representative will query on each subsequent visit as to the existence of the advance directive and whether any change has been made, or whether the advance directive has been revoked. Appropriate documentation will be entered into the medical record.

Requests to execute an advance directive:

1. Requests for execution of an advance directive will be forwarded to the patient representative department, which will follow the same process for documentation in the medical record as noted above.

References:

Joint Commission *Accreditation Manual for Hospitals*

Rights and Responsibilities of the Individual

RI.01.05.01, EPs 1, 4, 5, 6, 8, 9, 10, 11, 12, and 13

B.4 Sample Patient Complaints Policy

Policy name: Patient/family complaints
Policy number: 6
Written by:
Approved by:
Origin date:
Revision date(s):
Purpose: To establish a policy and procedure for patients and/or family to lodge complaints to the appropriate hospital authority and to have complaints reviewed and resolved

Policy:

The governing body is responsible for a timely and effective complaint resolution process. The governing body delegates the timely and effective complaint resolution process to the complaint resolution committee of the hospital.

Procedure:

1. At the time of admission or outpatient registration, the patient and/or family is informed of the complaint resolution process.
2. Information on the complaint resolution process is located in the patient handbook.
3. When possible, the manager of the unit/department should resolve the complaint as soon as feasible.
4. If the manager cannot resolve the complaint, he or she will seek direction from senior leadership, risk management, or the legal department.
5. If the complaint cannot be resolved immediately, the patient and/or family is informed that the complaint has been received and given a time frame for resolution of the complaint, which is not to exceed 10 working days from the date the complaint was received.

B.4 Sample Patient Complaints Policy *(cont.)*

6. The hospital provides the patient and/or family with the phone number and address of the appropriate state agency, The Joint Commission, and the state Quality Improvement Organization.
7. The hospital will allow the patient and/or family to voice complaints and recommend changes without coercion, discrimination, reprisal, or unreasonable interruption of care.
8. The hospital provides the patient and/or family with a written letter of the decision regarding the complaint. The written notice must include:
   - Name of the hospital contact person
   - Steps taken to investigate the complaint
   - Results of the investigation
   - Date of completion of the process

References:

Joint Commission *Accreditation Manual for Hospitals*

Rights and Responsibilities of the Individual

RI.01.07.01, EPs 1, 2, 4 6, 7, 10, 18, 19, and 20

APPENDIX C

Sample Informed Consent Form

Informed Consent Form for Operation/Procedure/Anesthesia/Transfusion

1. I give my permission to Dr. ____________________ (include any assistants) to perform the following procedure(s): ____

   ____

   ____

   on ______________________________ (patient's name).

2. I understand that during the procedure(s), new findings or conditions may appear and require an additional procedure(s) for proper care.

3. My doctor has discussed with me the items listed below:

   - The nature of my condition
   - The nature and purpose of the procedure(s) that I am now authorizing
   - The possible complications and side effects that may result, the problems which may be experienced during recuperation, and the likelihood of success
   - The benefits to be reasonably expected from the procedure(s)
   - The likely result of no treatment
   - The available alternatives, including the risks and benefits

   My physician has also explained that, in addition to the specific risks involved in the procedure(s), there are other possible risks that accompany any surgical and diagnostic procedure. I acknowledge that neither my physician nor anyone else involved in my care has made any guarantees or assurances to me as to the result of the procedure(s) that I am now authorizing.

Patient/guardian signature: ____

4. I know that other clinical staff may help my doctor during the procedure(s) and have been told of any surgical assistants that will assist my doctor.

5. I understand that the procedure(s) may require that I undergo some form of anesthesia, which may have its own risks. My doctor or a representative from the department of anesthesiology has informed me of the course of anesthesia that is recommended (if any) along with its possible risks and alternatives.

6. Any tissue or specimens taken from my body as a result of the procedure(s) may be examined and disposed of, retained, preserved, or used for medical, scientific, or teaching purposes by the hospital.

7. I understand that my procedure(s) may be photographed or videotaped and that observers may be present in the room for the purpose of advancing medical care and education.

8. I understand that during or after the procedure(s), my doctor may feel it necessary to give me a transfusion of blood or blood products. My doctor has discussed with me the alternatives to and possible risks of transfusion.

9. I understand what my doctor has explained to me and have had all my questions fully answered.

10. Additional comments: ____

____

____

____

____

Having talked with my doctor and having the opportunity to read this form, my signature below acknowledges my consent to the performance of the procedure(s) described above.

Signature of patient or legal representative ______________________________

Date __________________ **Time** __________________

Witness ______________________________

Date __________________ **Time** __________________

I have explained the risk, benefits, potential complications, and alternatives of the treatment to the patient and have answered all questions to the patient's satisfaction, and he or she has granted consent to proceed.

I have initialed the site with the patient and/or family for procedures that involve laterality or multiple structures, and/or levels.

Physician's signature ______________________________

Date __________________ **Time** __________________

